KW-363-223

The 28 Day Plan

GET FIT FOR SUMMER

Christine Green

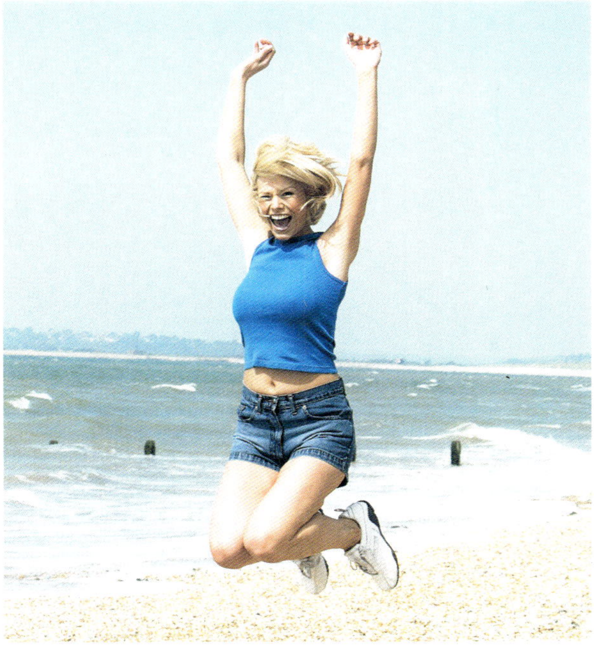

p

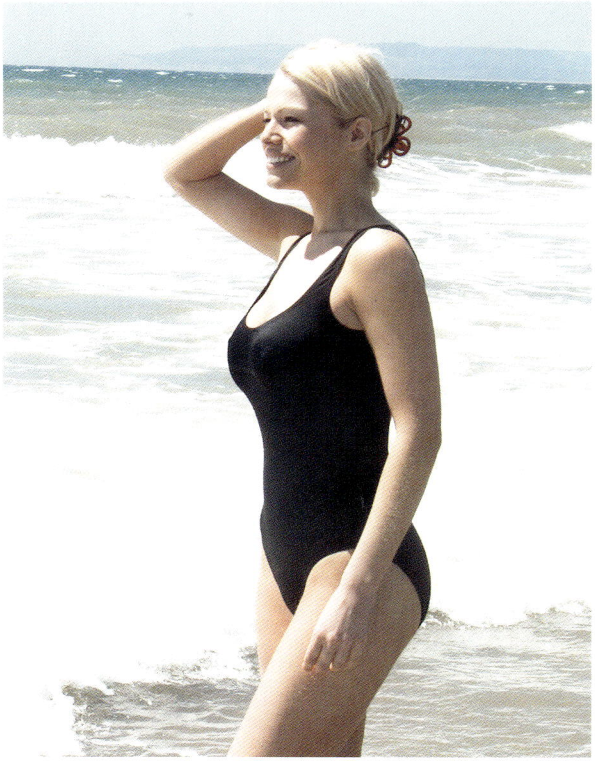

This is a Parragon Book

This edition published in 2002

Parragon
Queen Street House
4 Queen Street
Bath BA1 1HE, UK

Designed, produced and packaged by
Stonecastle Graphics Limited

Text by Christine Green
Edited by Gillian Haslam
Designed by Sue Pressley and Paul Turner
Commissioned photography by Roddy Paine

ISBN 0-75259-351-X

Printed in China

Disclaimer

The exercises and advice detailed in this book assume that you are a normally healthy adult. Therefore the author, publishers, their servants or agents cannot accept responsibility for loss or damage suffered by individuals as a result of following advice or attempting an exercise or treatment referred to in this book. It is strongly recommended that individuals intending to undertake an exercise programme and any change of diet do so following consultation with their doctor.

Contents

Get Fit For Summer

Are you ready for summer? Do you feel confident enough to cast off those long jumpers and baggy trousers and slip into something more revealing, or do you cringe at the thought of exposing your less-than-lean thighs and cower in embarrassment that you didn't do something about that slight bulge lying around your midriff before now?

Don't worry, help is at hand – if you follow this 28-day programme, you too can flaunt a well-toned body on the beach this summer.

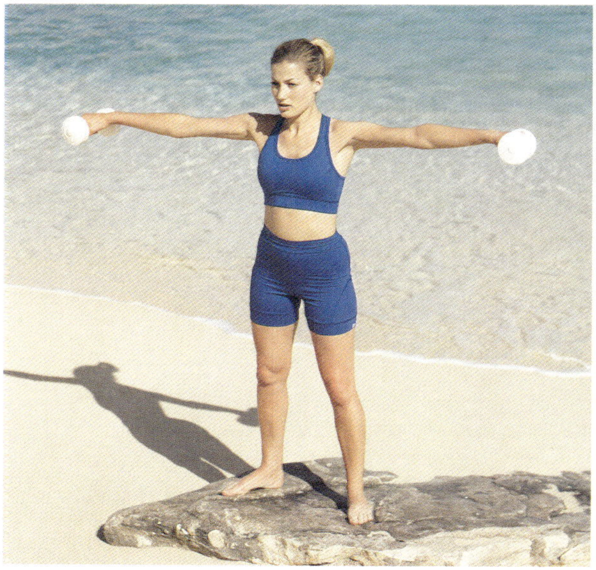

Are you fit?

Can you run upstairs without panting for breath? Take the family dog for a long walk and arrive home without feeling totally exhausted? Swim a couple of lengths at the local pool and not feel as though you had swum in the Olympics? If you can't, it looks as if you, along with many other people, are slightly unfit. However, the difference is that, simply by picking up this book, you have decided to do something about it.

Feeling fit and being fit are essentially two different things. We can't all afford the luxury of employing a personal trainer like some of the top stars to attain a wonderful sylph-like figure, but then again with a little time and effort on your part you can look just as good, if not better, even if it does entail having to forego that daily bar of chocolate or can of fizzy drink. But surely, at the end of the day, looking and feeling so much healthier is worth the initial input.

Feeling fit

Good health and feeling fit mean different things to different people. It could be the ability to do things that were impossible before, taking part in physical activities, feeling better about the way you look, feeling younger or feeling more active and alive when you wake up in the morning.

The essence of this 28-day programme is to illustrate that the secret of good health is a combined programme of healthy eating and exercise, changing bad habits for good habits, learning to listen to your body and making sure it remains at the optimum level of good health. So don't sit around poring over diet sheets; take time to work your way through this 28-day regime and find out for yourself what getting fit is all about.

WARNING
Before embarking upon this programme, it is wise to consult with your GP if you suffer from any of the following medical conditions:

- You are pregnant or breastfeeding
- You have diabetes
- Have anaemia
- Have diabetes
- Are underweight
- Are under stress
- Are taking medication that cannot be stopped

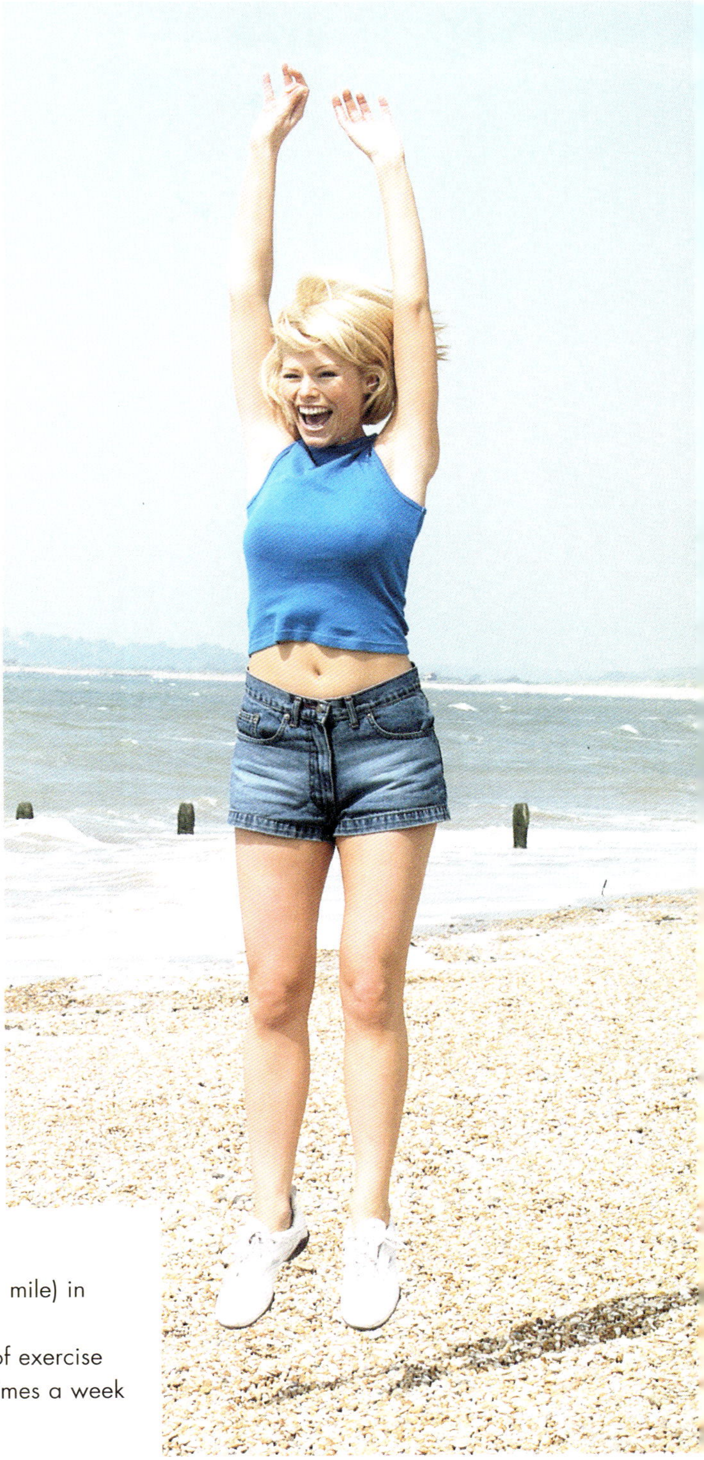

Before starting

If you are really serious, write out on a sheet of paper your reasons for wanting to get fit and set yourself some realistic goals to aim for but don't make them too extreme. Perhaps you want to go on holiday and wear a bathing costume for the first time in years, or feel confident enough to wear shorts during the summer; both are sound and reasonable targets that are achievable. When you feel fit, you automatically feel so much better about yourself, physically and psychologically:

When I get fit:

- I will look better on my summer holiday
- I will be able to wear a bathing costume
- I will be able to wear cropped tops
- My skin and complexion will look better
- I will feel more energetic and active

Did you know?

- You are technically unfit if you unable to walk 1.6km (1 mile) in 12 minutes without becoming out of breath
- If you want to get and remain fit the minimum amount of exercise required to maintain average fitness is 20 minutes three times a week

Assessing Your Diet

Do you follow a healthy, well-balanced diet? How much do you know about the food you eat? Do you read the labelling on the side of the packaging?

Did you know that at one time carbohydrate foods were the bad boys and therefore to be avoided at all costs, and yet recent research studies have revealed that a diet low in fat and high in carbohydrates is what we should aim for.

Nutritionists advise that in order for the body to function at its optimum it needs a well balanced diet which should include carbohydrates, protein, fats, minerals and vitamins. However, it is only by eating a variety of foods in sensible proportions that we can obtain the correct amount of nutrients needed to maintain good health.

The three basic rules regarding food are that:

1. It should nourish the body
2. Help safeguard health
3. Whenever possible play a role in helping fight against ailments or disease

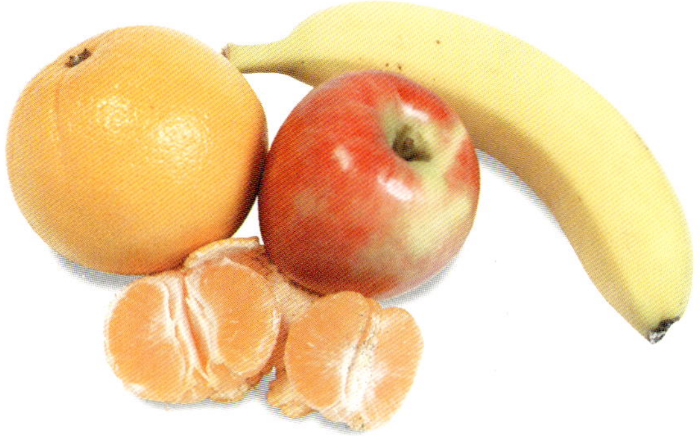

This programme is not intended as a weight-loss diet, although some people may find that they do lose a little weight, but rather a way of demonstrating to people a healthy way of eating.

How unhealthy is your diet?

How many times a week do you eat fish and chips or grab a burger at lunchtime? What about those pre-packed frozen meals that only require a blast in the microwave for several minutes or a meal in a can, that provides a meal within minutes?

The problem is that we live in an age where everything is needed yesterday, family meal times when everyone sits around the table together are fast disappearing and eating convenient 'fast' food often seems easier than choosing the healthy option. It is hardly surprising to learn that so many people are suffering eating disorders and allergies, so perhaps the time has come to take a look at our own individual eating habits.

Bad eating habits

- Skipping meals
- Eating junk and convenience foods
- Eating between meals
- Snacking on high sugary foods
- Eating when you are sad or worried
- Eating on the go

Skipping meals: one of the biggest problems when people are in such a hurry is that they find themselves skipping meals, so they may have breakfast then not eat anything until later in the evening, surviving on a diet of coffee and a chocolate biscuit.

Convenience foods: we are a nation of fast-food junkies in that anything that is quick to prepare is fine to eat, hardly giving its nutritional value any consideration. Although ready-prepared meals do save time this doesn't prevent them losing valuable nutrients during reheating, and experts have found that convenience foods contain more sugar, salt and fat than most other foods. However, to counterbalance the argument, it must be said that there are an increasing number of 'healthy' or 'calorie-counted meals' now available.

Fast foods: the occasional burger or meal of take-away fish and chips is fine provided it is not a diet based purely on fast foods. Although certainly of a higher quality than ten years ago, the fact is that most do contain a lot of calories and a lot of fat.

Eating between meals: most people do snack between meals; for many with little or poor appetites this is the ideal way for them to maintain their energy levels. But problems occur when snacking is largely confined to sugary or salted foods, cream cakes or crisps. If you do snack between meals, then think healthy and choose from the following list:

- ✓ Apples
- ✓ Bananas
- ✓ Handful of dried fruit
- ✓ Oranges
- ✓ Pears
- ✓ Celery
- ✓ Raw carrot
- ✓ Cauliflower florets

And remember, if you are a snack eater the frequent presence of food in the mouth can encourage the build up of bacteria that in turn cause plaque, so brush and floss the teeth regularly.

Eating when sad: many people turn to food when they are angry or sad, depressed or worried, even on some occasions when happy, but there is always an underlying factor to trigger this behaviour. It could be you have just ended a relationship, lost your job or feel under stress and food is your only ally. But when it results in putting on extra kilos when you'd much rather prefer not to, then it becomes an enemy. So if you find that you are always nibbling for no particular reason, try to find out the cause before it gets out of control.

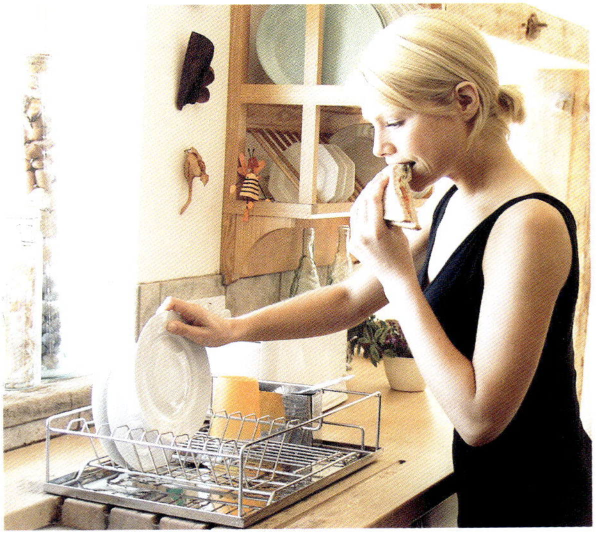

Eating on the go: never eat on the go. It's not healthy and it doesn't give the body time to digest the food. So if you find you are guilty of this, the simple answer is to stop!

Good eating habits

It is possible to adopt good eating habits and although it may seem you are having to give up all the things you enjoy eating, you are wrong. It doesn't mean having to forgo eating a cake or a packet of crisps, eat them by all means, just in moderation. Instead of having three glasses of wine when you go out, have one. When the family is having an apple pie and custard for their dessert, skip the apple pie and just have an apple. And if you fancy a bar of chocolate, then have the occasional small one.

Good eating habits

- ✓ Eat three balanced meals a day
- ✓ Don't snack on sugary foods
- ✓ Don't deprive yourself of everything you enjoy

What Does A Healthy Body Need?

In order to function at its optimum a healthy body needs a well-balanced diet which should include carbohydrates, protein, fats, minerals and vitamins.

Carbohydrates: the main function of carbohydrates is to provide energy for the body. During digestion carbohydrates are converted into glucose and then absorbed into the bloodstream. It is the glucose that the body uses for energy. If energy is not immediately required, it is stored in the muscles and liver as glycogen and is readily available to be converted into glucose when extra energy is required. Foods containing carbohydrates include: sugar, syrup, jam, honey, fruit, bread, puddings, cereals, potatoes.

Proteins: these are invaluable to the body for their vital role in repairing and maintaining the tissue, muscles and blood cells. An excess intake of protein is either converted into energy or transposed into fat and held in the body for emergency use. Found in foods including: meat, fish, cheese, eggs, milk, soya beans, nuts, cereals and pulses.

Fats: the role fats play in the body's energy status is to supply it with a concentrated source of energy and also essential fatty acids, vital for maintaining healthy skin and the regulating body functions. Found in foods including: milk, butter, cream, cheese, suet, fatty meat, oily fish, margarine, salad or cooking oils.

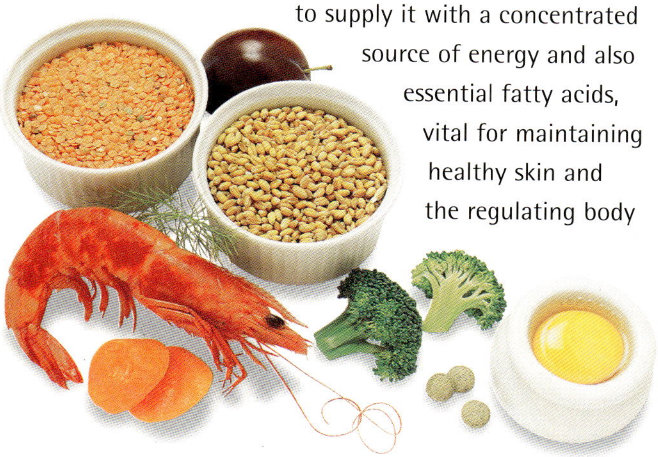

Vitamins: important for healthy functioning of cells. Present in small amounts in all foods, a varied, sensible diet including a high proportion of fresh fruit and vegetables will ensure a sufficient intake for good health although some vitamin loss occurs during cooking. Foods containing high levels of vitamins include fresh fruit and vegetables, milk, butter, cheese, eggs, margarine, fish.

Minerals: inorganic substances found in foods from both animal and vegetable sources and required in very small quantities. They are essential for the repair of tissues, healthy formation of bones, teeth and blood cells, maintenance of body fluids and metabolic functions. Foods high in mineral content include dark green leafy vegetables, sardines, liver, kidney, egg yolk, yogurt, milk and cheese.

Achieving a balanced diet

Health authorities in Britain and the United States have drawn up guidelines for healthy eating. There are five identified by the British Health Education Authority, whilst six appear in the four-tier US food pyramid. The American pyramid differs from the British model only in that it places fruit and vegetables into separate categories. The other four groups are shared by both and include the following:

Six daily servings of complex carbohydrates.
Including bread, cereals, potatoes, pasta, rice and noodles.
• Choose wholemeal brown or high fibre breads, increase your intake by making thicker sandwiches but with less filling. Eat bread with main meals and have a larger helping of potatoes, rice or pasta rather than higher fat foods.
• Don't fry any of the foods in this group.
• Don't spread butter or margarine thickly on bread.
• Don't add cream or rich sauces or oily dressings to these foods.

Five daily servings of fruit
This includes fresh, frozen and canned fruits, fruit juice and dried fruit.
• Select a wide and varied range of fruits and have more than one as a dessert by making up a bowl of fruit salad. Add fruit to a sandwich filling. Make a fresh fruit or vegetable drink.
• Don't, however, eat excessive amounts in one sitting as this could lead to indigestion.

Five daily servings of vegetables
This includes all types of vegetable.
• Use tomatoes and other vegetables, fresh or frozen, in sauces or serve as a traditional side dish or with meat or pasta.
• Don't deep-fry vegetables – they will soak up the oil.
• If stir-frying, do so in a little oil which is healthier.

Two daily servings of milk and dairy products
This includes semi-skimmed milk, cheese, yogurt, calcium-enriched soya milk.
• Eat only moderate amounts, choosing reduced fat versions such as semi-skimmed milk or low-fat yogurt (always check the labelling before buying).
• Don't consume large amounts of full-fat varieties of cream, milk, cheese or butter.

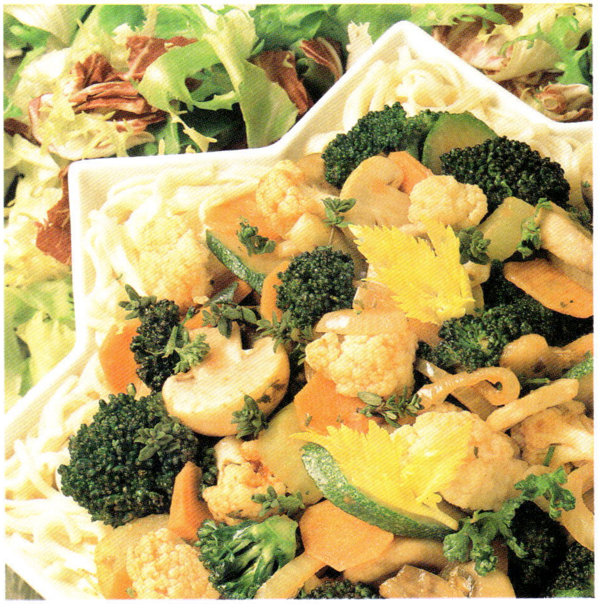

Two daily servings of protein
This includes oily fish, lean meat, chicken, turkey and fish.
• Eat moderate amounts of these foods, choosing only those that are lean with all visible fat trimmed. Try eating fish at least twice a week and include some oily fish such as mackerel or salmon.
• Don't fry meat or fish.
• Don't add fat to those already rich in oils. Instead grill, poach, steam, stir-fry or even roast – all are healthier cooking methods.

Two daily servings of fats
This includes margarine, butter, chocolate, crisps, biscuits, pastries and sweets.
• Choose lower fat brands or eat only small amounts, using spread and oils sparingly. Skim any fat from meat juices when making gravy.
• Don't be tempted to eat more than one chocolate or fill yourself up between meals with sugary snack foods or high fat snacks such as crisps.

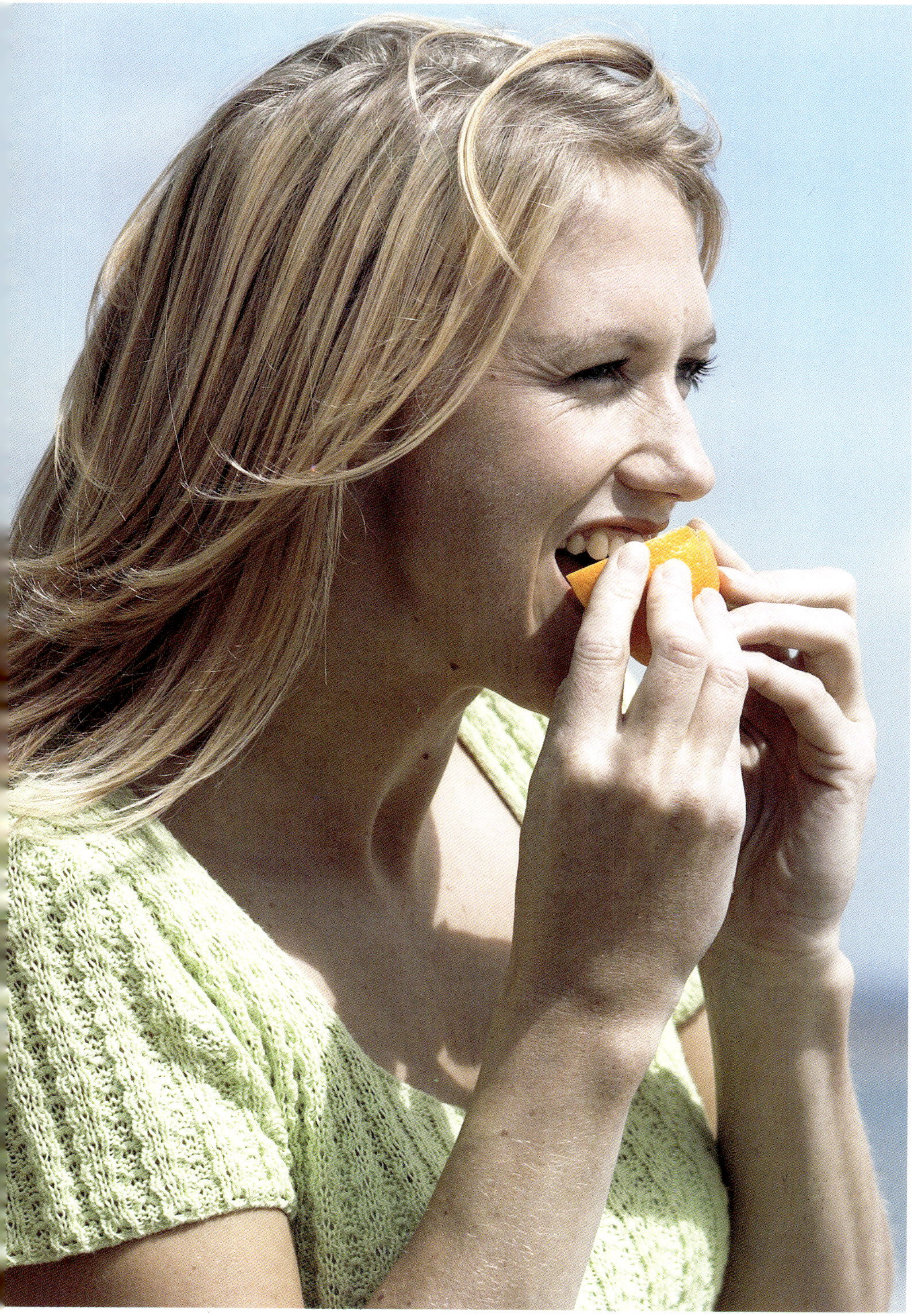

Little treats

You can eat as much fruit as you like – it's a convenient snack food, packed full of goodness and available in many different shapes, sizes and flavours.

But we all need a little extra sweet treat now and then:

Bread and jam: there's nothing like a slice of bread and jam and you can still indulge, provided you chose wholemeal bread and choose a low-sugar jam.

Chocolate: in moderation chocolate can be healthy. It can provide a good proportion of an adult's daily copper intake,- necessary to help create red cells and strengthen bones.

Cheese: nutritious but some varieties are high in fat and should be eaten in moderation. But if you enjoy eating cheese with a meal, try those with a lower fat content such as cottage cheese, ricotta or fromage frais.

Ginger and carrot cake

2 teaspoons ground ginger
175g (6oz) dark brown soft sugar
225g (8oz) self raising flour
2 large carrots, washed and grated
1 egg, beaten
250ml (8fl oz) skimmed milk

Preheat the oven on to 190°C/350°F/gas mark 4. Line a 450g (1lb) tin with greaseproof paper. Blend the ground ginger, sugar and flour into a bowl. Add in the grated carrots and stir. Add the egg to the milk and stir this into the mixture, blending in well. Pour the mixture into the prepared tin and bake in the oven for approximately 55 minutes, or until a skewer inserted into the cake comes out clean. Leave to cool.

Healthy eating tips

This programme isn't about losing weight, nor is about calorie counting. It is about looking at ways to eat healthily and curb any bad eating habits you may have adopted over the years.

- Drink lots of sparkling water – it fills you up, keeps you hydrated and helps flush waste products from your body. Aim for at least 8 glasses a day.
- Don't overeat – get into a habit of eating slightly smaller portions and if you still feel hungry, wait 10 minutes before returning for a second serving.
- Eat plenty of plant-based foods such as fruit, grains and vegetables as they're packed with nutrients. Include lean protein foods too, but only low-fat dairy products in small amounts.
- Habits are difficult to break but it isn't impossible. Eating on the go or, worse still, eating from the bag is hardly going to do your digestive system much good. So make a rule to only eat at the table with a knife and fork.
- Don't drink your calories – chewing takes longer and ultimately provides more satisfaction. Instead of drinking a glass of orange juice, why not eat an orange instead?

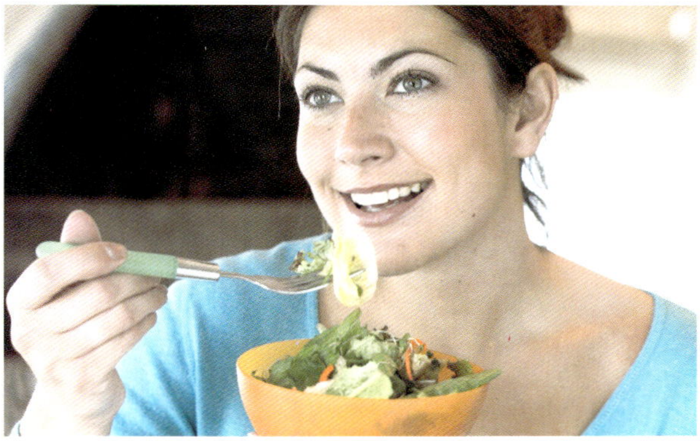

When following this 28-day programme:

- Eat regularly and enjoy your meals
- Eat a wide variety of foods
- Eat enough to maintain your weight and height
- Eat plenty of foods rich in carbohydrate and fibre
- Don't eat too much fat
- Don't eat sugary foods too often
- People with special dietary requirements and those under medical supervision should check with their GP to see if this balance of foods is suited to them.
- If you drink alcohol, keep within the sensible limits
- Use only moderate amounts of salt in cooking and don't add salt to your meal
- British nutritionists recommend we should drink 1.5-2 litres (3-4 pints) of fluid a day to maintain health liquids. Most of this should be made up of water.
- Ensure you get plenty of vitamins and minerals in your diet (perhaps take a supplement each day)

Healthy Meals

If you are looking for some tasty meals for your new eating routine, here are some suggestions you may like to try.

Breakfasts

- Bowl of muesli with fresh fruit, followed by a slice of wholemeal toast with a little butter or low-fat spread and marmalade.
- Bowl of cornflakes topped with a grated apple and served with skimmed or semi-skimmed milk, plus a glass of fresh unsweetened orange juice.
- Bowl of cornflakes with several strawberries and skimmed or semi-skimmed milk
- Two slices of wholemeal bread filled with grilled lean bacon
- One poached egg on a slice of toasted wholemeal bread

Haddock omelette

This is great for the weekend when you have more time to prepare a special breakfast.

3 egg whites
Salt and pepper
Spray bottle of light oil
50g (2oz) smoked flaked haddock
1 small tomato
2 slices of wholemeal bread

Whisk up the egg whites and season with salt and pepper. Spray a shot of light oil into a non-stick frying pan and, when it is heated through, pour in the egg mix. Shake the pan well and cook the egg whites. Remove the pan from the heat, and add the flaked haddock, then pop them under the grill for 3 minutes. Meanwhile, halve the tomato and grill it. Toast the bread. Turn the omelette onto a plate and serve with the wholemeal toast and the tomato.

Kiwi smoothie

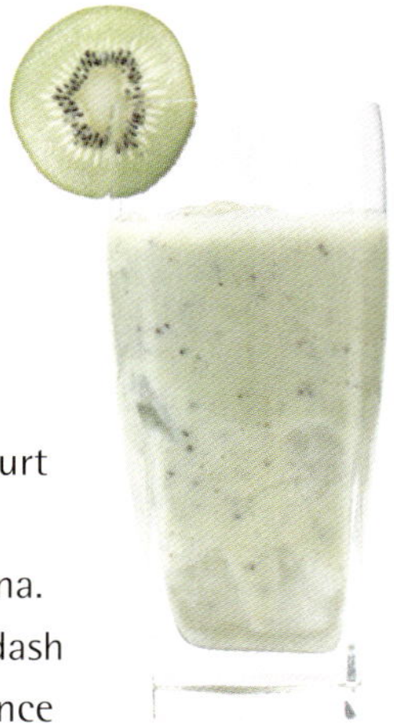

A treat for those who prefer to drink their gourmet breakfast.

4 kiwi fruits
1 small banana
Lemon juice
Small carton low-fat natural yogurt

Peel the kiwi fruits and the banana. Add them into a blender with a dash of lemon juice and the yogurt. Once blended, pop some ice into a glass and pour the smoothie over.

Lunch

If you have the time here are some ideas for nutritious lunchtime recipes you can try. Some of them could be prepared the evening before and stored in the refrigerator.

Mackerel toasties

Something to rustle up in a few minutes. Drain a can of mackerel fillets and put them into a bowl. Mash them up with a fork and stir in a teaspoon of mustard and some chopped spring onions. Lavishly spread the mixture over two slices of wholemeal toast and pop under the grill for a few minutes until warm.

Drumstick supreme

A very easy recipe which makes a tasty lunchtime treat.

1 clove garlic, peeled and crushed
1 teaspoon dried oregano
1 teaspoon dried thyme
1 teaspoon dried rosemary
25g (1oz) breadcrumbs
Salt and pepper
4 chicken drumsticks
2 tablespoons low-fat natural yogurt

Pop all the ingredients, except the drumsticks and yogurt, into a plastic bag and give it a good shake. Using a very sharp knife carefully pierce the drumsticks then cover liberally with the yogurt. Pop the drumsticks into the bag and give another good shake, making sure they each get well covered with the ingredients. Remove from the bag and place each under a pre-heated grill for approximately 15 minutes, turning them once. The drumsticks are ready to eat when no pink juices trickle out when pierced with a skewer.

Spanish omelette

A delicious lunchtime snack that can be served hot or cold.

1 tablespoon olive oil
1 medium onion, peeled and sliced
1 clove garlic, peeled and crushed
$^{1}/_{2}$ pepper, red, green or yellow
450g (1lb) new potatoes, cooked and diced
4 eggs, beaten
Salt and pepper

Pour the tablespoon of olive oil into a frying pan and sauté the sliced onion and garlic. When just turning golden brown, add the potatoes. When browned, add the eggs, salt and pepper and cook slowly until firm.

Spicy chicken

This is the ideal lunchtime dish when you have friends calling around, as the quantities will serve four.

1 large chicken, cut into four pieces
Salt and pepper
1 teaspoon curry powder
Pinch of celery salt
$^{1}/_{2}$ teaspoon ground ginger
150ml (5fl oz) low-fat natural fromage frais
1 teaspoon paprika

Wash the chicken and season the inside with salt and pepper. Mix the curry powder, celery salt and ground ginger together, then add it to the fromage frais. Place the chicken in a microwave-proof dish. Pour the fromage frais mixture over the chicken and then sprinkle with paprika. Pop it into the microwave on high for 8 minutes per 450g (1lb). Leave it to stand for 15 minutes before serving. The chicken is ready to eat when, pierced with a skewer at the thickest part, the juices run clear; if still pink then cook for a little longer and test again.

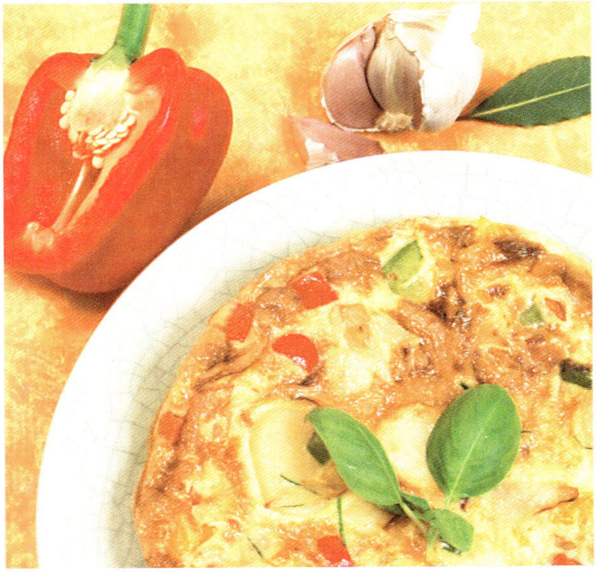

Dinner

Mealtimes can a problem when you run out of ideas, but there are lots of delicious meals you can prepare with a little thought and ingenuity that will appeal to all the family.

Chilli con carne

A great family dinner, serving four.

450g (1lb) lean minced beef
1 large onion, peeled and chopped
400g (14oz) can chopped tomatoes
2 bay leaves
1 teaspoon Bovril
425g (15oz) can red kidney beans
1 teaspoon chilli powder
2 cloves garlic, peeled and crushed
Black pepper

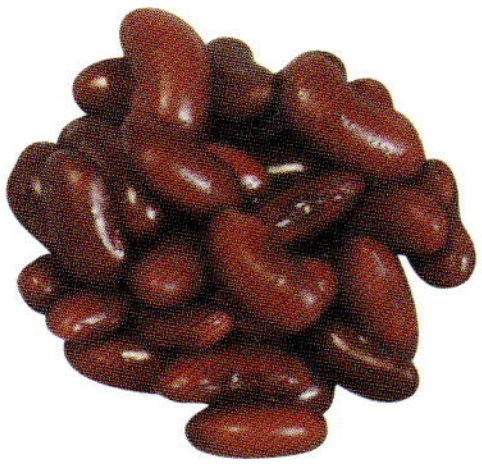

Dry-fry the mince in a non-stick frying pan, then drain it through a colander. Clean any fat from the frying pan, then add the onion and dry-fry it. As the onion is turning brown, return the mince to the pan together with the tomatoes, bay leaf, Bovril, kidney beans, chilli powder and garlic. Season with black pepper. Cook for about 10 minutes, stirring occasionally and adding a little water if it becomes too thick. Serve with brown boiled rice.

Chicken celebration

Serves four.

Black pepper
4 chicken breasts, skinned
225g (8oz) brown rice
450g (1lb) canned beansprouts
Soy sauce

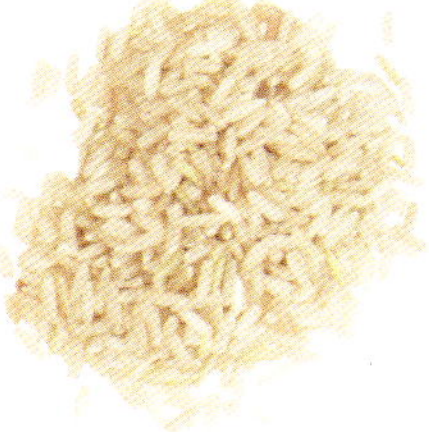

Sprinkle a preheated non-stick frying pan with black pepper, then add the chicken and sauté until it begins to turn brown. Generously sprinkle the chicken pieces with more black pepper before turning over on to the other side to cook. Cover the pan with a lid, turn the heat down slightly and leave the chicken gently simmering for a further 20 minutes, checking every 5 minutes or so and turning the chicken over to cook on the other side.

Whilst waiting for the chicken, cook the rice in boiling water and drain. Pop the rice and drained can of beansprouts into a colander and pour a kettle of boiling water over to reheat them. Drain and tip onto a serving dish, placing the chicken pieces on the top and adding an extra tang with a dash of soy sauce.

Chicken risotto

Serves four.

25g (1oz) low fat spread
225g (8oz) skinless chicken, cut into small bite sizes
1 green pepper, de-seeded and finely chopped
1 small onion finely chopped
1 clove garlic, crushed
Herbs to season
700ml ($1^3/_4$ pt) chicken stock
275g (10oz) long grain brown rice
1 tablespoon lemon juice
275g (10oz) mushrooms, sliced
Tomato slices to garnish

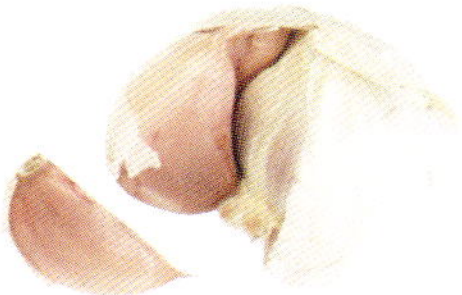

Melt the low fat spread in a large pan and add the chicken, pepper, onion, garlic and seasoning. Cook for 5 minutes. Add the stock, rice and lemon juice continue cooking with the lid on over a medium heat for 20 minutes. Add the sliced mushrooms and cook for a further 5 minutes. Serve garnished with slices of tomato and a mixed green salad.

Strawberry sorbet

Healthy, nutritious and a perfect source of Vitamin C.
450g (1 lb) fresh strawberries, washed and hulled
Juice of 1 large orange

Put the strawberries into a food processor with the orange juice and blend. Pour the mixture into a bowl and pop into the freezer for 1 hour. Remove and leave it to thaw slightly, then beat with a metal spoon and return to the freezer for a further 5 hours. To appreciate the taste, the sorbet should be left to soften at room temperature for 20 minutes before serving.

Melon delight

450g (16oz) melon
275ml (10fl oz) low-fat flavoured yogurt
225g (8oz) green grapes

Chop up the melon flesh and separate it equally between 4 tall glasses then spoon generous amounts of yogurt over the top. Cut the grapes in half and share them between the glasses. Spoon the rest of the yogurt over the top and pop into the freezer to chill.

If you feel peckish at any time during the day, avoid that tempting chocolate bar or packet of crisps and eat a low calorie snack of healthy fruit or vegetables. Choose from:

- An orange
- Handful of grapes
- Handful of cherries
- Cauliflower florets
- A stick of celery
- An apple
- A banana
- Dried fruit
- A carrot
- A pear

Desserts provide the finishing touch to a delicious meal but avoid eating anything too heavy. Try the following ideas:

- 1 meringue nest filled with 115g (4oz) fresh fruit and topped with 50g (2oz) low-fat yogurt
- 2 pieces of fresh fruit
- Diced apple and pear with low-fat yogurt

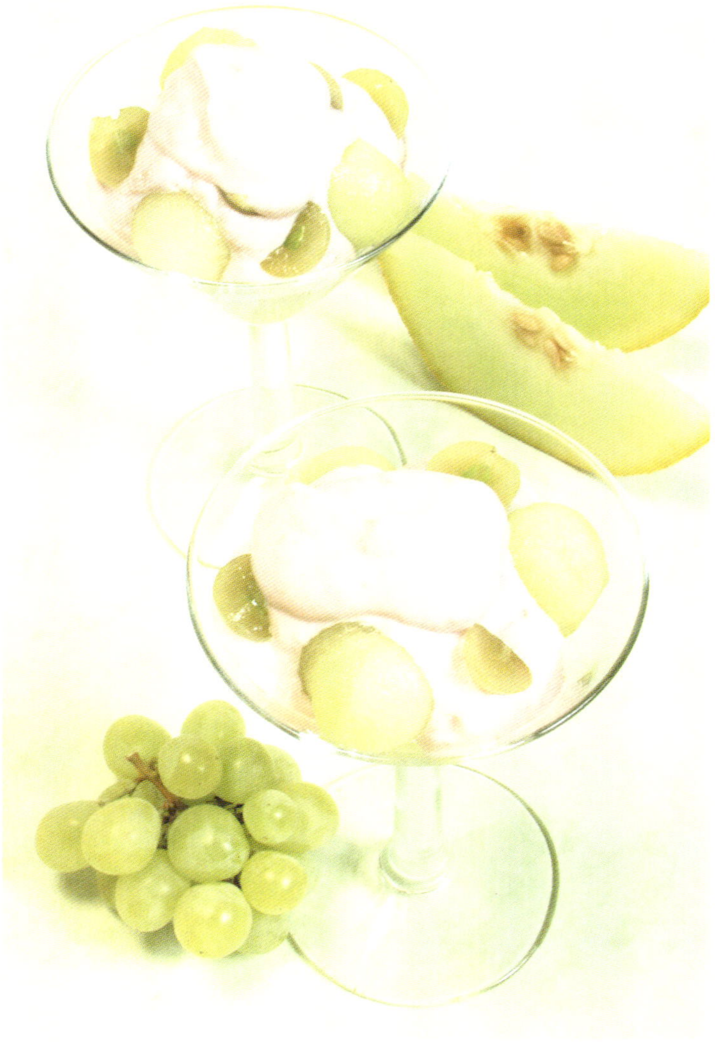

Daily Exercises

There are four main reasons why most people become bored with exercising: lack of time, no local gym, boredom, absence of results.

Lack of time: if you really want to do something, you will make time for it. And just imagine how much benefit you will gain from exercising – you will feel fitter and healthier, have a reasonable level of fitness and be better equipped to deal with stress. Besides, you don't have to take part in a marathon or go jogging – exercising can amount to a brisk walk, doing some gentle workout exercises at home, or even gardening.

No local gym: there's no need to enrol at a gym – you could rent a keep fit video or go for a swim at your local pool.

Boredom: this is a popular excuse, or is it just an excuse for opting out? There are lots of ways you can make exercising more fun – exercise at different times of the day, ask a friend to join in or work out to some music. You could also enrol at an activity class at your local college.

Absence of results: if you set yourself small goals and then keep a diary recording what you have achieved and how you feel, you will then spot those small changes that may have otherwise gone unnoticed.

Before you begin your new programme

If you have recently given birth, have been inactive for several years or suffer from any of the medical conditions listed below, then you should, for your own safety, consider making an appointment to see your GP before beginning an exercise routine.

- High blood pressure
- Heart trouble
- Family history of early stroke or heart attacks
- Frequent dizzy spells
- Extreme breathlessness after mild exertion
- Arthritis or other bone problems
- Severe muscular, ligament or tendon problems
- Other known or suspected disease

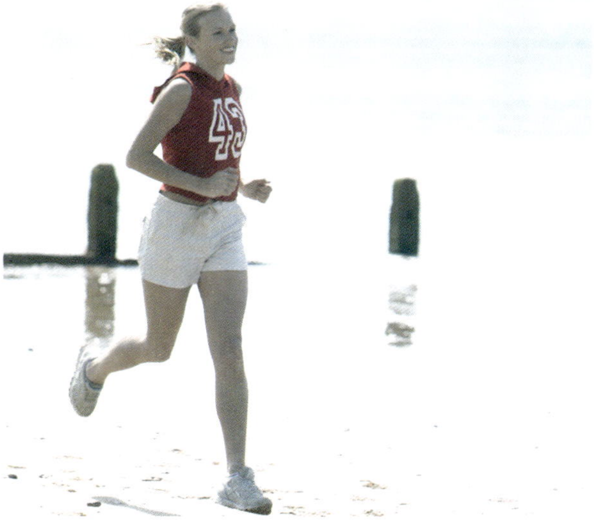

Exercises for specific areas of the body

There are exercise routines to help tone up all parts of the body and if you have one particular area that you feel needs more work than another, then simply spend more time working on that. But if you are looking for an all-round tone up exercise regime, try this routine every day which takes approximately 20 minutes. Make sure that you drink plenty of water.

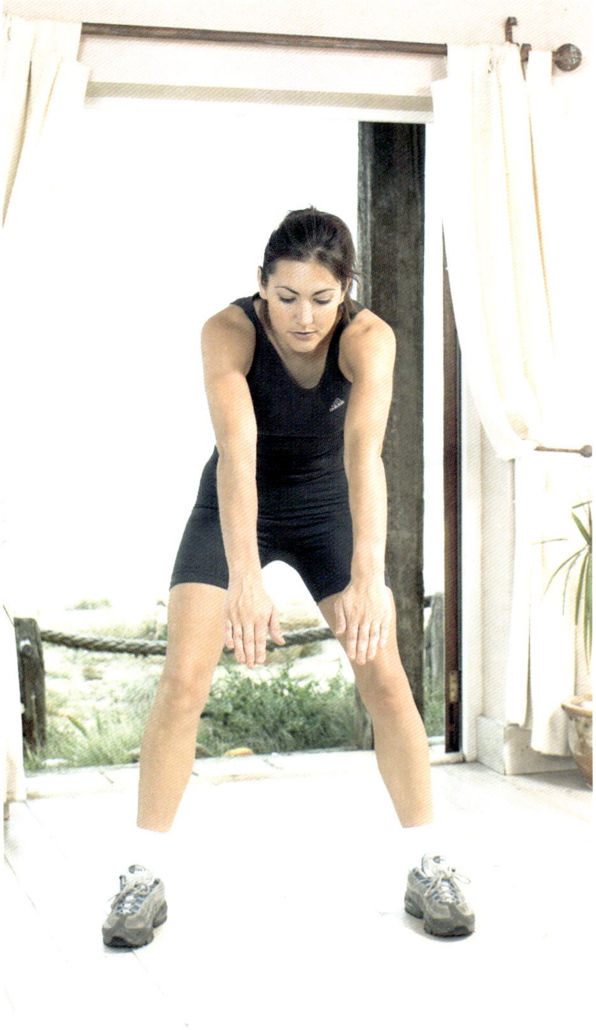

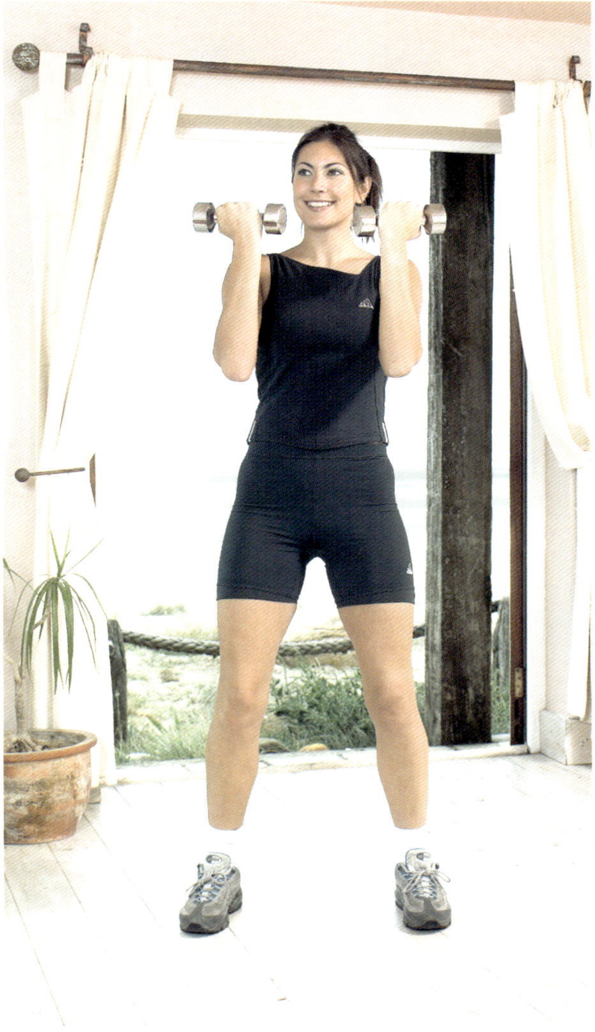

Warm up

It is essential before any workout routine to spend 5 minutes warming the muscles up.

1. Stand with the feet apart and swing the arms forward and down between your legs, bending the knees as you do but keeping the back straight.

2. Straighten your legs, swing your arms back up to the stretched position.

3. Inhale as you stretch, and exhale as you curl down.

4. Repeat as fast as you can 20 times.

Arms and chest

An ideal exercise for trimming upper arms and lifting the chest.

1. Stand with both feet hip width apart and arms down by your sides, holding a light weight (such as a can of beans) in each hand.

2. Bring the arms slightly forwards, raise the hands, then bend and lift the elbows up and back, pushing hard.

3. Lower the arms back down and repeat 30 times.

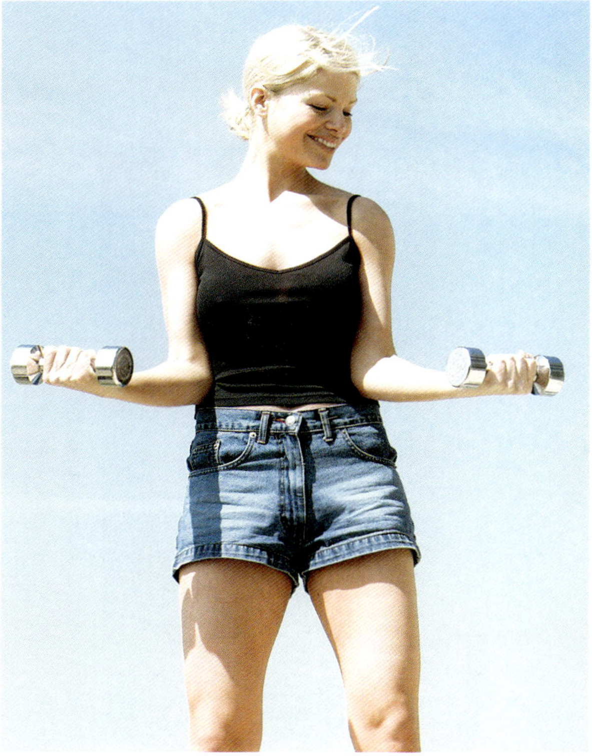

Stomach and waist

1. Stand with feet hip width apart, arms down by your sides and still holding on to the weights, raise the arms to shoulder level, then bend the elbows.
2. Punch the right hand hard to the right, twisting the body round at the same time so the hips are front-facing.
3. Return to the standing position and this time punch your right fist to the left, twisting the body around as much as possible. Repeat 20 times.
4. Repeat the same sequence but this time with the left hand. Repeat this 20 times.

You may find it more comfortable if you use a thin workout mat for the floor exercises.

Thighs

This tones and strengthen thigh muscles.

1. Stand with feet hip width apart and hands resting on the hips.
2. Put the right leg forward and bend the knee, with the left leg back and knee bent, almost touching the floor.
3. Jump into the air, crossing the legs so the right leg comes forwards and the left leg goes back.
4. When landing, allow the knees to bend then jump and cross the legs over again.
5. Repeat 20 times.

Stomach

1. Lie down on the floor, with hands by your sides, both palms facing down and feet together.
2. Slowly raise both legs vertically.
3. Lower the right leg almost to the floor, then as you begin to raise it again, lower the left leg almost to the floor. Both legs should cross in a scissor position.
4. Repeat 10-20 times.

Hips, buttocks and legs

1. Continue lying on your back on the floor, arms spread horizontally, palms down.
2. Raise the left leg as high as possible, making sure it is kept perfectly straight.
3. Move the foot towards you, cross the leg over to touch the floor on your right side, reaching as high up your body as you are able to. Keep legs straight and shoulders touching the ground.
4. Repeat with your right leg in the same way.
5. Repeat 10 times.

Cool down

Lie on the floor, relax and rest for one minute, allowing your body to cool down and your heart rate to return to normal.

Other exercises

If you feel you really haven't the time to spend 20 minutes on a workout, then just do what you are able to.

Exercises for the middle body

This is ideal for working on those flabby abdominal muscles.

1. Lie on your back with knees bent and feet hip width apart on the floor.
2. Bend your elbows and place your hands behind your ears so that your fingertips touch.
3. Move your chin so it is in alignment with the rest of your spine and move your elbows slightly inwards.
4. Pull in your abs gently towards your spine.
5. Curl slowly upwards and forwards until the head, neck and shoulders are clear of the floor. Hold that position for a count of ten, then slowly lower and then repeat.

For the back area

1. Lie on your stomach, arms and legs outstretched.
2. Tilt your head forward so it is resting on the floor or, if more comfortable, rest it on the side.
3. Lift your right leg and right arm a few centimetres off the floor and stretch them out towards opposite ends of the room.
4. Hold for one minute, then slowly lower them back down to the starting position.
5. Repeat with the other arm and leg.

For shoulders and arms

1. Kneel on the floor with your weight in your hands.
2. Pull in your abs so that your back doesn't sag.
3. Bend your elbows and lower your body down towards the floor.
4. Once your upper arms are almost parallel with the floor, press back up to the starting position, hold and then repeat.

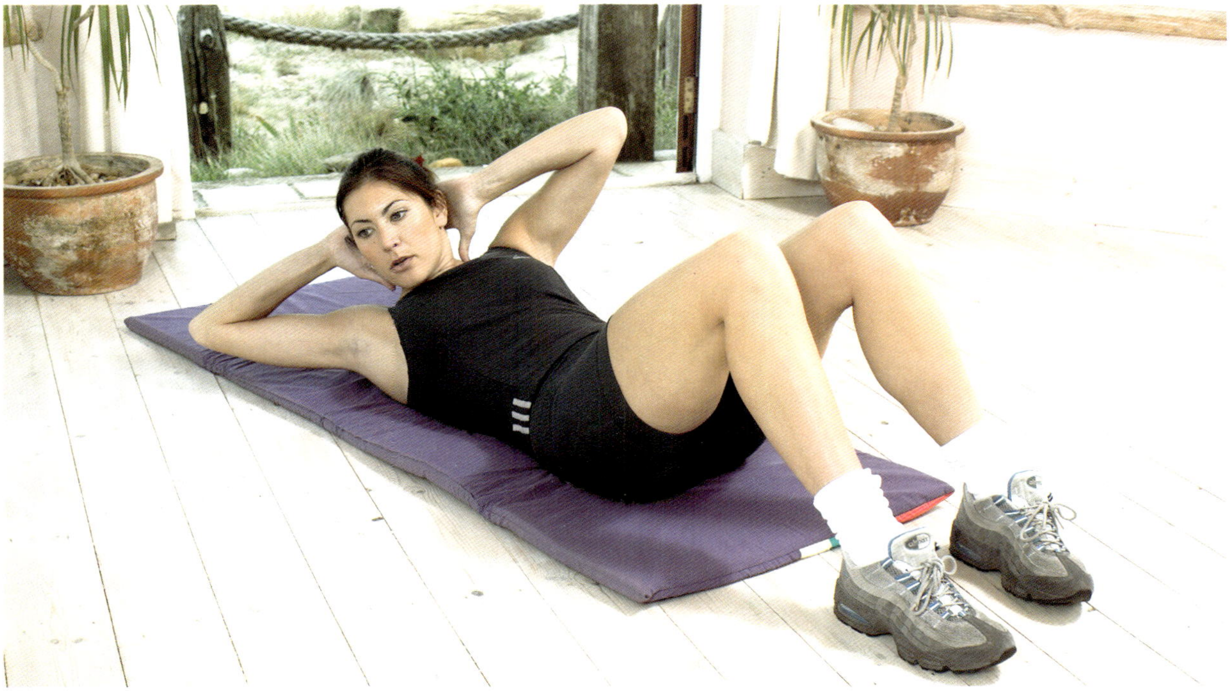

Exercises for the reluctant keep-fitter

If you have been working all day, then possibly the last thing on your mind is doing anything more physical other drinking a cup of tea. But it is still quite possible to tone and trim muscles even when sitting on the sofa.

Head

Look directly in front and extend the back of the neck up and towards the ceiling whilst easing the shoulders down, keeping your jaw parallel with the floor. Hold for 5 seconds and repeat the other side.

Shoulders

Ease both shoulders forwards and upwards, then back and down. The secret is to move through each new direction in one continuous circle, say it out loud: forward, upwards, backwards, downwards, making the circle as large as you are able.

Waist

1. Sit upright on a chair or stool with legs and feet hip width apart, knees directly over the ankles.
2. Put your arms at chest level, bent at the elbows with forearms resting on one another.
3. Twisting from the middle, slowly turn your head shoulders and arms around to the left as far as possible, keeping your shoulders down throughout this move.
4. Return to the starting position and repeat the other side.

Energetic exercising

Exercise that makes you sweat a little is perfect for the battle of losing weight and is known as 'aerobic' exercise, covering any activity that you can do for long periods of time. Your own personal level of fitness will partly determine the type of exercise you take part in, but it is important not to push yourself. Go at your own pace and increase your workout gradually. If you feel ill, dizzy, faint or in any way poorly, you must stop any exercise and check with your GP before taking it up again.

The main aim is to work out for 20-40 minutes each time, building up gradually, as you become fitter. Alternatively, break your sessions up into 10-minute routine. The long-term effect of exercise is that you will build up the amount of muscle in your body and decrease the amount of fat. The more muscle you have, the more food you are able to eat without gaining weight.

Fact

Every 450g (1lb) of muscle in your body burns off 35 calories a day.

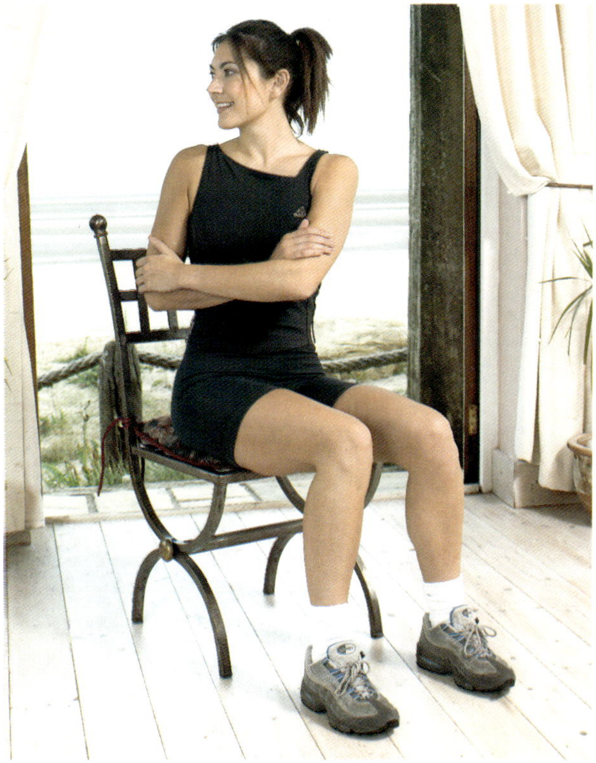

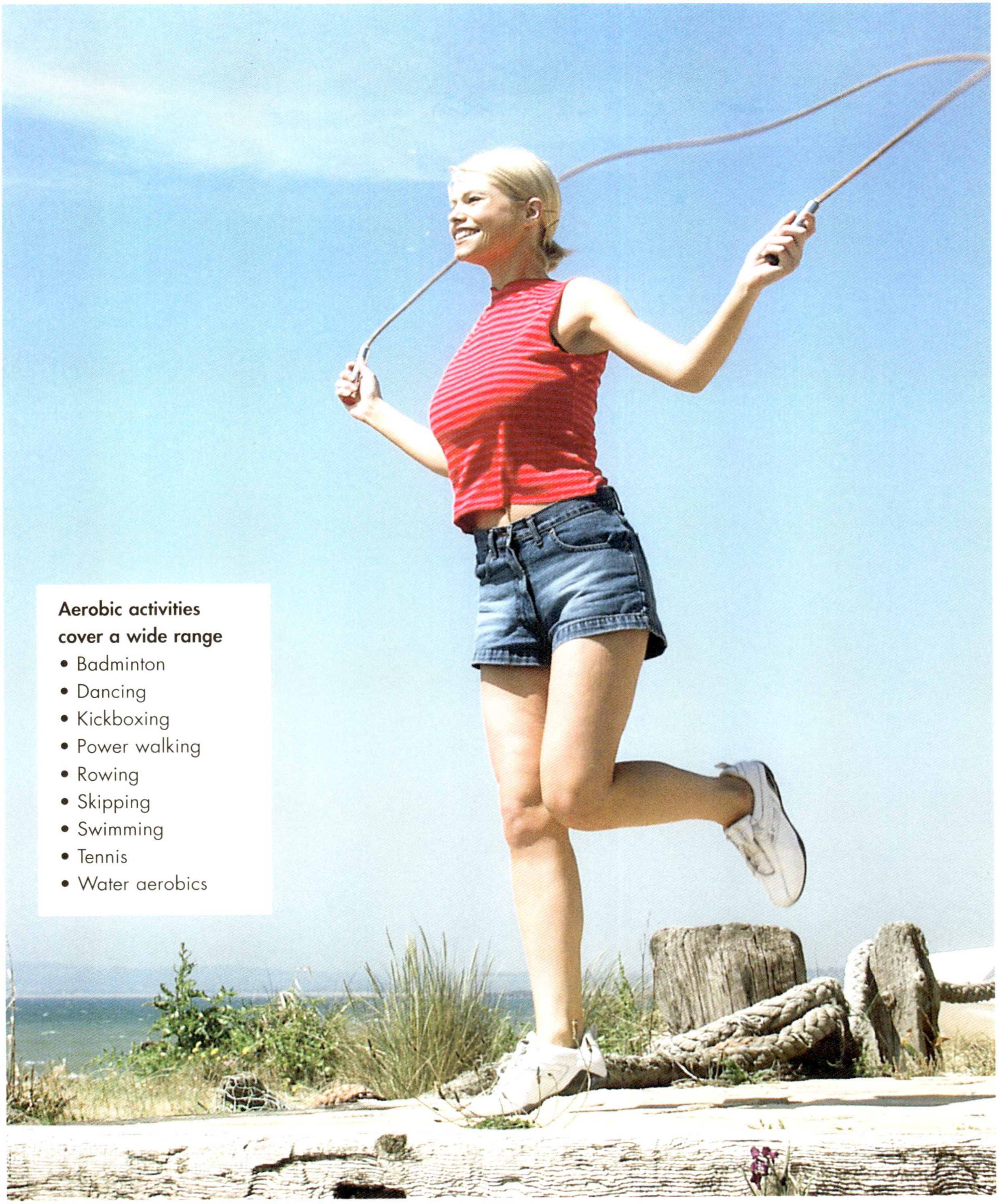

Aerobic activities cover a wide range

- Badminton
- Dancing
- Kickboxing
- Power walking
- Rowing
- Skipping
- Swimming
- Tennis
- Water aerobics

Daily Treatments

To achieve ultimate success on the programme – a healthier, fitter body – it is important that you include each of the following treatments in your 28-day plan.

Daily treatments

- Start the morning with a drink of hot water with a dash of lemon juice
- Take a daily energy shower
- Spend 30 minutes exercising
- Take a brisk 30-minute walk
- Spend 20 minutes in hibernation

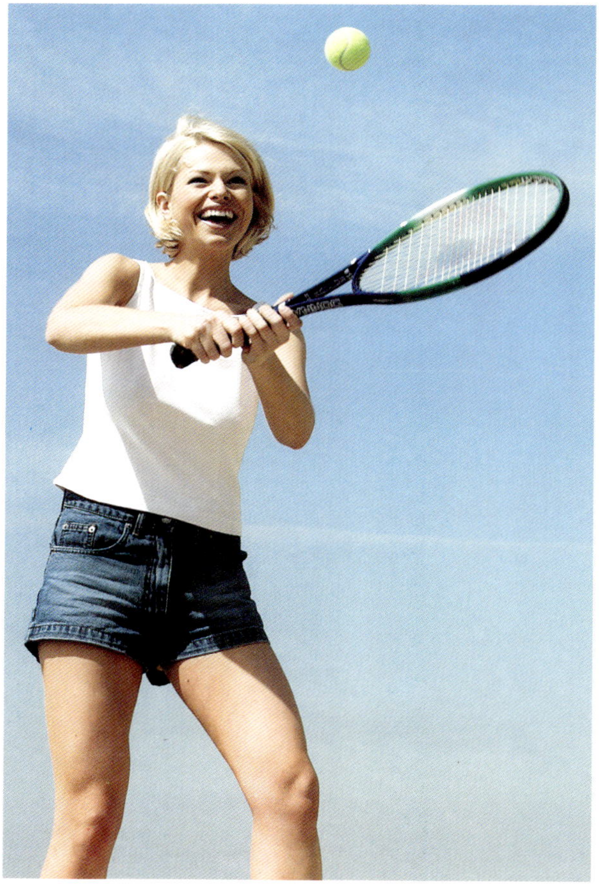

Extra treatments

- Every week give yourself a salt scrub
- Every three days have a salt bath

Hot lemon water: begin the day with a hot cup of water and a squeeze of lemon/lime juice. This will freshen your mouth and is good for helping to cleanse the system.

Energy shower: there's nothing like an early morning energy shower to kick-start the body into action, so the first thing each morning jump into the shower and, if brave enough, when you are ready to come out, turn the cold tap full on for several minutes.

Exercise to energize

Keep these three words firmly focused in your mind's eye. Write them in large print on a piece of paper and pin it up in the kitchen or bathroom so whenever you feel sluggish you can remind yourself.

If you haven't exercised since the day you left school, apart from walking to the shops, then you are bound to feel a little apprehensive. But all the experts advocate that a daily dose of activity helps our emotional and physical wellbeing and actually increases energy levels by releasing endorphins which are the body's natural high hormones and make you feel great. When you first begin exercising, take it easy – don't overdo it and gradually build up. By the end of the programme exercising will form part of your daily routine.

Walk

Make a determined effort each day to go for a walk, even if it is just to the shops. Try to walk for at least 20-30 minutes because walking:

- Helps stabilize blood sugar levels and therefore helps to avoid mood swings
- Can alleviate stress, tension and depression due to those 'feel-good' hormones it triggers
- Is an ally against the development of osteoporosis because it is a weight-bearing exercise
- Combined with healthily eating there is no better way to help fight the flab
- Strengthens the heart
- Speeds up mental alertness
- And can even help and cure back pain by building up the muscles that stabilize the spine

Hibernation

It is amazing how a daily 20-minute mini-break can restore depleting energy resources and recharge flagging batteries. Just take yourself off somewhere, perhaps to a quiet room or out in the garden, where you can feel totally relaxed and allow yourself to 'switch off' for 20 minutes. Think about no one and nothing but peace and tranquillity.

Body scrubs

In order to improve the skin's texture and tone it up, body scrubs are well worth including in the programme and should ideally be undertaken either before or during a shower, as they can be rather messy.

They involve massaging the skin with a gritty substance to remove dead skin cells and engrained grime and improve the overall appearance of the skin. They can either be used on their own or with a rough flannel or loofah to increase their effectiveness.

Body scrub recipe: For an inexpensive scrub mix a handful of sea salt with a dollop of olive oil, leave for

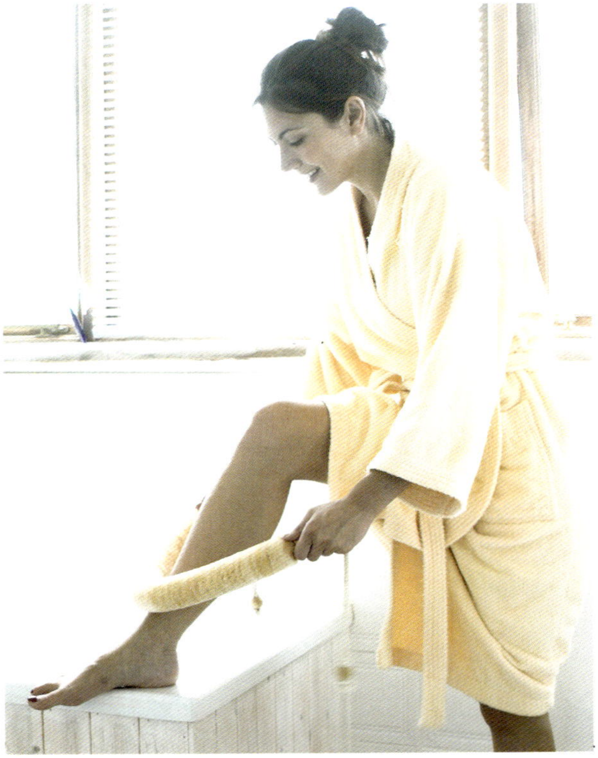

a few minutes to give the salt time to dissolve slightly, then rub it all over the body and rinse off.

Salt bath

Bathing in a solution of Epsom salts is good for the skin as it draws out toxins through the pores. Run the bath water and add 225-450g (1/2-1lb) of Epsom salts. Soak for about 20 minutes, and when you get out, keep yourself warm by piling on lots of clothes. This will help the body to continue sweating out the toxins.

Don't be surprised if you are feel thirsty afterwards – it is the effect of sweating which causes this. Just make sure you drink lots of water.

Salt baths are not advisable if you have:

• Heart or kidney problems • High blood pressure

Maintaining The Programme

Often the most difficult part in following any programme is preventing boredom from setting in. This is why it is important to integrate some little treats into your programme.

Do something totally wild and out of character – spend an afternoon at a funfair and relive your childhood days, book yourself on a bus trip for a day, surf the net, call up an old friend, have a wardrobe or make-up blitz and get rid of all your old clutter to make way for the new you.

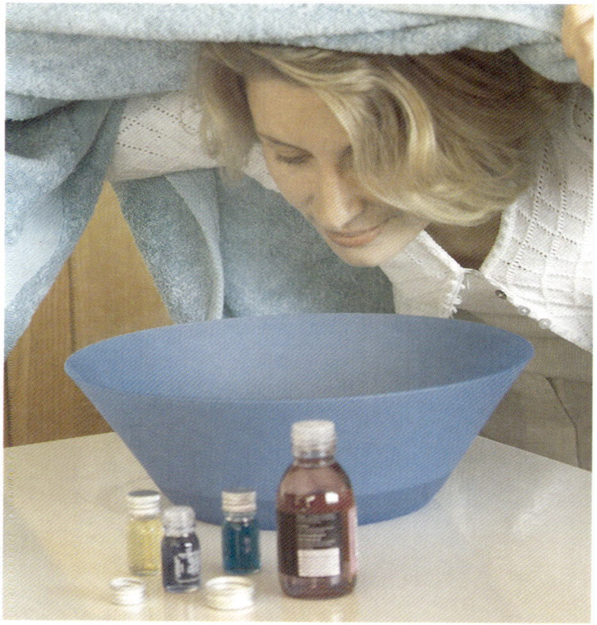

Think calm

We all get days when we feel totally stressed and agitated, but a few minutes spent relaxing can calm away those tensions and frustrations and help you put things into perspective. One useful trick is to inhale essential oils. Fill a large bowl with boiling water and add two drops each of clary sage, rosemary and geranium essential oils. Lean your head over the bowl (not too close or you risk scalding yourself) and trap the steam by draping a towel over your head. Now close your eyes and breathe deeply for 5 minutes.

Rest

During part of the day, if you feel particularly stressed or anxious for no apparent reason, try to take yourself off somewhere peaceful, go into another room and listen to some calming music or do a short relaxation exercise.

- Sit in a comfortable position, close your eyes and breathe in through your nose.
- Feel the breath reach deep down into your lungs.
- Exhale slowly through your mouth and remain still for a few moments listening to the sound of your breath.
- Become aware of your body relaxing.
- Begin with the muscles of your scalp and face and slowly work down your body, releasing all the tension as you go.
- Concentrate on your favourite colour and then picture it in its brightest form. Imagine it turning darker, then visualize it dancing around and creating patterns.
- Slowly allow the colour to drain away and watch as it becomes paler and paler until eventually it disappears.
- Disregard any thoughts that may creep into your mind whilst concentrating, brush them aside and keep firmly focused on your colour.

Meditation and relaxation aren't always easy to master but they are worth the effort. Several minutes of inner silence on a regular basis will provide you with an experience to last a lifetime. Make time each day to relax and relieve the tensions in your body and allow your mind to be free from daily worries. Don't force yourself – if at first it doesn't work, wait a couple of days and then try again.

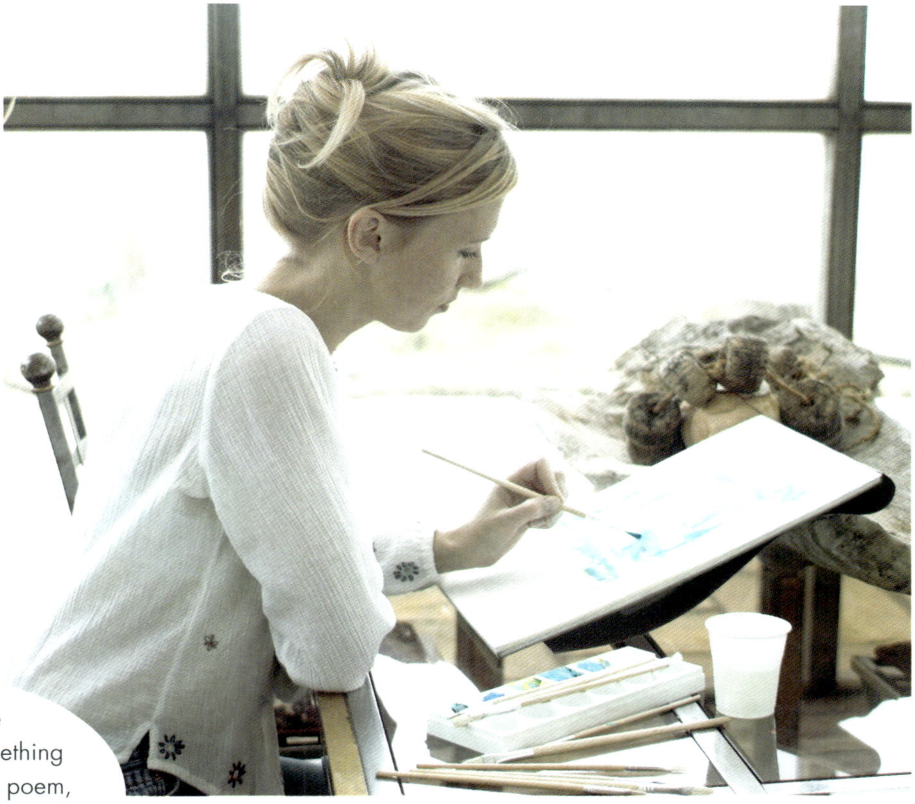

Be creative
Why not do something creative – write a poem, paint a picture, write a letter to a friend.

Singing

Many people who suffer from panic attacks find that singing loudly makes them feel better. Singing helps you breathe more deeply, giving your body the oxygen it needs to get you back in control.

Blitz the make-up

With a new healthier lifestyle and a trimmer body, surely the time has arrived to throw out some of your old make-up. Spend an afternoon at the local beauty section of your department store where the staff are always willing to give you advice on the best colours or shades to suit your skin. Some will give you a free make-up too.

Exfoliate the skin

The skin cells generally renew themselves every 3-4 weeks, but as you get older this process slows down and you can end up with a dull, lifeless complexion. Using an exfoliating cream or gel once or twice a week clears away those dead skin cells to leave your skin cleaner, brighter and fresher.

Splash warm water over your face and dab the exfoliator cream on your forehead, nose, cheeks and chin and then begin slowly massaging it around your face using small circular movements. This is perfect for boosting the circulation, but avoid the delicate areas around the eyes. Don't forget the neck.
Rinse off with lots of warm water and then finally a splash of cold water. Pat your skin dry with a soft towel and apply a moisturiser.

Get Fit: Days 1–7

Okay it's here; you've done all your preparation, and you know what the next 28 days will involve. The best and most effective way to undertake the programme is to start on a positive note and preferably on a Friday, thus giving you the weekend to get into some sort of routine.

Whether you are a working woman or a busy mum at home, the next 28 days may mark the biggest changes you are ever going to make in your life so be prepared. Make up a chart (see page 31) and stick it on your kitchen wall so that you remember what you must include each day in your programme.

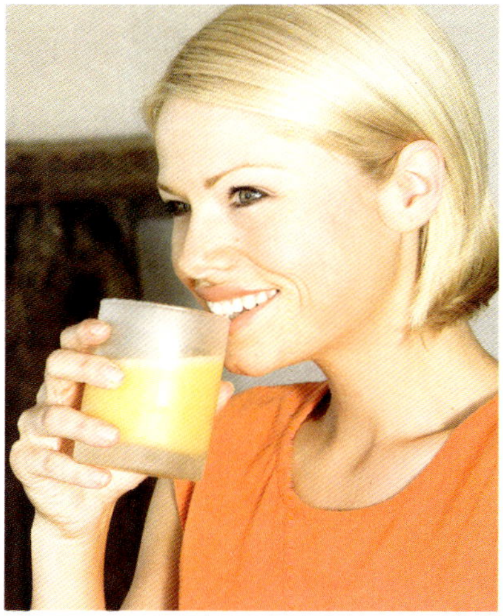

It's important to keep a diary in which you can record your day's plan, what you ate, how you took time out for yourself, and then at the end of each day make a note of how you felt. Obviously some days you will find more to write about than others, but keeping this and then referring to it when you have negative days will keep you motivated. Weigh yourself today only!

Here is a typical plan for day one, but naturally times will differ and the order in which activities are done may also change according to your lifestyle.

7.30am Glass of hot water and squeeze of lemon juice.
7.45am Early morning shower
8.15am Breakfast. On the first day choose something you are familiar with, such as cereal, to ease you gently into the programme.
9.15am After clearing away the breakfast dishes, begin day one with a gentle body workout but take it easy and don't over exert yourself.
10.15am Sit down and relax with a glass of water and don't think too hard about those parts of your body that may be aching at the moment. The next time will be better. Whilst you are sitting, why not practise 20 minutes of hibernation to give your body time to settle down.
11.00am Although you are on the programme, don't forget there is always the housework to do and in fact if you put sufficient energy into doing this you will be burning up even more calories.
1.00pm Time for lunch. For a healthy sandwich, take two medium slices of wholemeal bread and fill with low-fat spread, a small can of tuna in brine, a few lettuce leaves, a small tomato and several slices of cucumber. Finish off with a banana.
3.00pm Go out for at least a 30-minute brisk walk. You'll tone up your legs and buttocks and, if you take long strides, your lower tummy muscles will benefit too. Set yourself a goal and see if you can achieve it.
4.00pm Make yourself a cold drink of freshly squeezed

orange juice to revive you after that long walk. Why not take the opportunity to make this your creative part of the day when you can dedicate it to doing something artistic – paint a picture, write a poem or take up tapestry or embroidery.

6.00pm Time to think about dinner – why not prepare a chicken salad, taking advantage of the variety of salad vegetables around. And if still peckish afterwards, have some fruit.

7.00pm Have an early bath. Add some salts into it and relax for a while.

8.00pm Snuggle into your dressing gown and before going to bed, spend some time thinking calm thoughts to relax your mind and prepare you for a good night's sleep.

Don't forget – as you complete each activity tick it off on your chart and before you go to sleep remember to record in your diary how you felt, both the good and bad points. Plan what you intend doing the next day.

Remainder of the week

The remainder of week one should follow more or less the same basic routine, but adding in different foods and trying different exercises

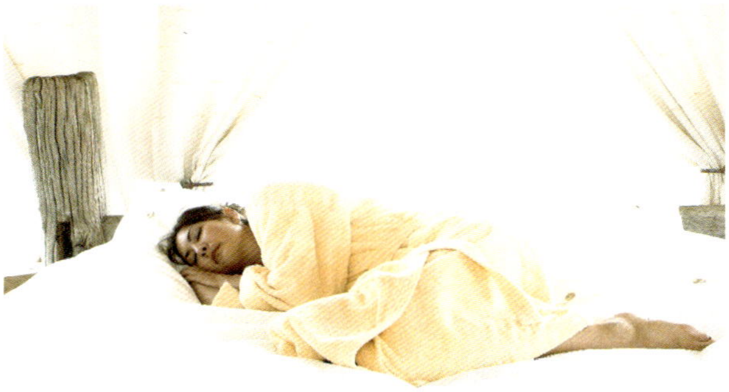

It's a good idea to keep an exercise diary to record your increased stamina and fitness. For example:

Date	Exercise	Repetitions	Comments
01.04	Crunches	20	Agony!
	Hips/Buttocks	30 each	Breathless
02.04	Stomach	20	Exhausted
	Swimming	30 mins	Tired but feel great
03.04	Hips/Buttocks	40 each	Much better today
	Stomach	30	Puffed - easier today
	Walking	2 miles	Brisk and energizing
04.04	Crunches	30	Getting much easier

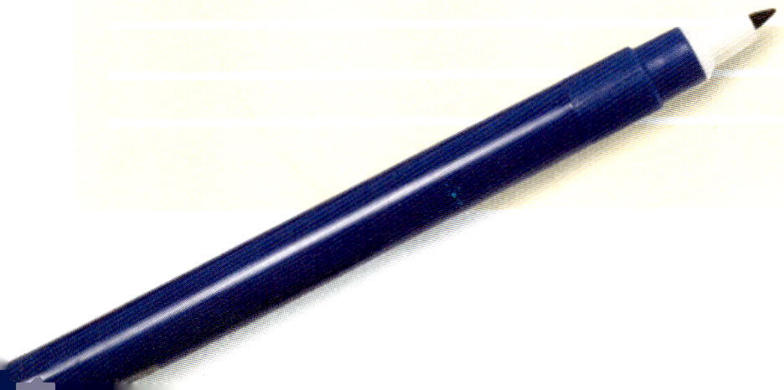

Measurements chart

As you change your routine to include more exercise and reform your eating habits, you will find that not only will you have toned up the muscles all over your body to give you a slimmer look, but you will feel generally a lot healthier and have lots more energy!

You can record your measurements each week using this simple chart.

	Week 1	**Week 2**	**Week 3**	**Week 4**
Date				
Weight				
Bust				
Waist				
Hips				

Get Fit: Days 8–14

You will by now have established a routine and perhaps made some changes.

So are you ready for week two?

7.30am Glass of hot water and squeeze of lime juice.
7.45am Early morning shower.
8.15am Breakfast. Have a change in your second week – why not try a poached egg on wholemeal toast.
9.15am By now you should have extended your target for walking and so be able to walk a little further.
10.15am After the walk your feet may feel a little tender so why not treat them to some pampering that will help make them feel nice and smooth. See the recipe for Foot Mask, below.
11.00am Make this your creative time and carry on with the picture you were painting or the tapestry you began and to make it more relaxing play some music in the background.

Foot Mask
2 bananas
2 teaspoons olive oil
2 tablespoons fine sea salt
Juice of half a lemon

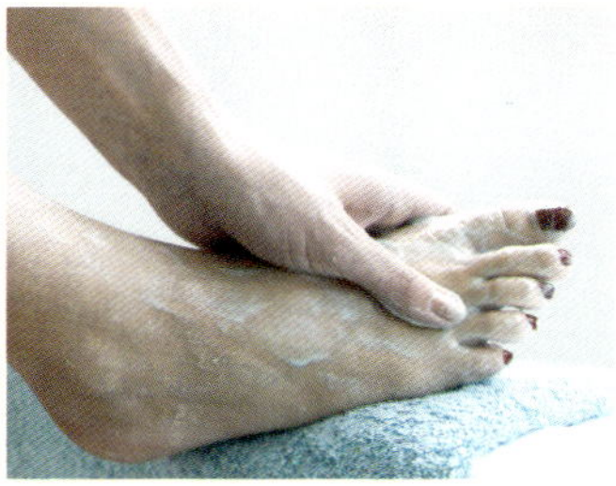

Mash the bananas in a bowl, then add the rest of the ingredients. Mix them thoroughly. Place the feet on a towel and massage the mixture into them. Leave it on for about 10 minutes and then wash off using warm water. Afterwards apply lots of moisturiser.

1.00pm Time for lunch. Often the worst time of the day as you try to think up tasty meals. This is why it's a good idea to work out a week in advance what you intend eating and stick to those meals. Write them up as a daily menu and pin it in the kitchen. Today why not have a baked jacket potato filled with a small can of mixed chilli beans and served with a green salad.
3.00pm Do a total workout routine.
4.00pm Spend time exfoliating the skin
6.00pm Time to prepare dinner. How about Chicken Risotto and finish with a banana for dessert.
7.00pm Go into a quiet room and spend some time hibernating to help clear your mind of all tensions and frustrations. Just being alone for 20 minutes can help to revitalize and rejuvenate the body.
8.00pm Treat yourself to a relaxing bath and give those muscles a long, lingering soak by adding a few drops of sweet marjoram, ginger or black pepper oil to the bathwater.

Don't forget – as you complete each activity tick it off on your chart and before you go to sleep remember to record in your diary how you felt, both the good and bad points. Plan what you intend doing the next day.

Remainder of the week

Just continue keeping to more or less the same routine you have already established but add in different foods and try out different exercises. Pamper yourself with a salt bath.

Get Fit: Days 15–21

You are now beginning the second half of your programme and into the third week already.

There may be times you become bored with doing the exercises or toning up routine, but you are doing it for a good reason so just keep on and reap the rewards in another week!

7.30am Glass of hot water with a squeeze of lemon or lime juice.
7.45am Morning shower.
8.15am Breakfast. A bowl of muesli with a handful of dried apricots and bananas and some skimmed milk. Cup of herbal tea.
9.15am Try to do the full workout – by now you should be able to do far more of each routine. Look in your diary to check on your progress.
10.15am Arrange to meet up with an old friend and leave the house earlier so you can go for a walk beforehand. If you feel you are in need of some support with your workout routine, why not call in to your local gym and check whether they have any classes you could join.
12.00pm Have lunch with a friend. Perhaps choose a chicken salad and a glass of iced water.
2.15pm Back at home it's time for a little rest and hibernation.
3.00pm Do some housework or perhaps some gardening. The grass needs mowing and some plants need pruning, and there is also weeding to be done.
4.15pm Time for a glass of unsweetened orange juice and an hour of creative inspiration.
6.00pm Prepare dinner – Chicken Celebration tonight.
7.00pm As a treat, bake a Ginger and Carrot Cake.
8.00pm Have a salt bath, then an early night. Record what happened during the day and plan the following week's menus.

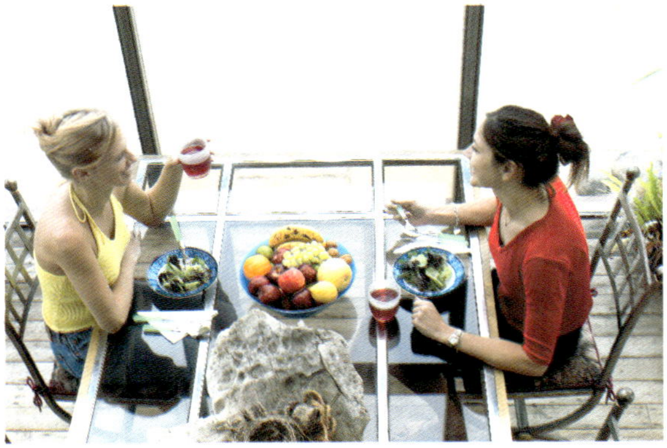

Don't forget – as you complete each activity tick it off on your chart and before you go to sleep remember to record in your diary how you felt, both the good and bad points. Plan what you intend doing the next day. Why don't you take some photographs of yourself midway through the programme just to see what you looked like at different stages.

Remainder of the week

By now you will have established a pattern of exercising and also the creative hour to spend however you wish. You can always alternate and change things around, you may even find that you want to replace walking with something entirely different. The number one priority is that you stick to the programme.

Get Fit: Days 22–28

You are on the last lap. This is the final week and you have come a long way so there is no turning back now. The end is actually in sight.

Once you hit the age of 30-40 you've got to be careful about activities that involve pounding. Running takes its toll on the joints but swimming improves the metabolism and cardiovascular fitness; tones you from head to toe and it's also a great calorie burning activity. Start with 20 minutes and if you can do five lengths of the pool, next time see if you can do six lengths, gradually building it up.

7.30am Have a glass of hot water with a squeeze of lemon juice.
9.15am Instead of doing your usual exercise i.e. walking or cycling, why not go for a swim at your local pool. An invigorating early morning swim is healthy and refreshing and it sets you up for the rest of the day.
10.15am Breakfast. A wedge of melon served with 115g (4oz) grapes and a small carton of low-fat yogurt.
11.00am Swimming can be refreshing but also tiring so give yourself a little time and do some relaxation.
1.00pm Lunchtime. How about a Spanish Omelette.
2.00pm Creative hour.
3.30pm You should by now have increased the length of your workout sessions so prepare yourself and start pumping those muscles.
5.00pm Have a cool glass of water with a slice of lemon and sit down to think over your month's busy schedule and what you have achieved, what you would like to have achieved and feel very proud of what you have done
7.00pm Go out for a celebration meal. Whatever restaurant you go to, choose your menu wisely – you don't want all that good work going to waste.

Now is the time to weigh yourself and take your measurements, then look back at the beginning of the chart to see the amount of weight you have lost.

Here are some suggestions for meals that won't ruin all your good work:

If eating French
- Crudités with garlic dip (raw sliced vegetables)
- Moules Marinières (mussels cooked in shallots, lemon, herbs and white wine)
- Steak au Poivre (steak with a peppered sauce)

If eating Italian
- Minestrone soup (made with white beans, peas, onion, ham, celery, herbs, garlic, pasta and white wine)
- Spaghetti Napoli (pasta with a low-fat tomato sauce)

If eating Greek
- Spanokopitta (pastries stuffed with feta cheese and spinach)
- Souvlaki (pieces of meat marinated in olive oil and lemon juice then grilled on skewers)
- Greek Salad (sliced tomatoes, onion, black olives and lettuce with feta cheese)

If eating Spanish
- Gazpacho (cold soup with red peppers, onions, tomatoes, cucumber soaked in oil, garlic and vinegar)
- Arroz alla Alicantina (rice with chicken)

Activity Record Chart

Record your activities every day using this table

DAILY ACTIVITIES	1	2	3	4	5	6	7	8	9	10	11	12	13	14	15	16	17	18	19	20	21	22	23	24	25	26	27	28
Glass of hot water and lemon or lime juice																												
Daily energy shower																												
Breakfast																												
Lunch																												
Dinner																												
1.75 litres (3 pints) water																												
Wide variety of fresh fruit																												
Wide variety of fresh vegetables																												
30 mins walk																												
30 mins exercise																												
20 mins hibernation																												
Epsom salts bath every 3 days																												
Salt scrub once a week																												
Only moderate use of salt																												

Congratulations!

You've done it – you've completed the 28-day Get Fit for Summer programme successfully.

But old habits are hard to break and just as there have been moments in the last 28 days when you felt unable to go on, there are sure to be days in the future when you feel like going back to your old ways and not thinking about what you are eating. When you get moments like those, read back through your diary to remind yourself how you coped with those down days. Look through the photographs you had taken at different stages of your programme and glean from them the confidence to continue.

And it is worth remembering that different stages of life can create their own problems:

In Your Twenties – welcome the office bum.
This is when many of us end up sitting at a desk for 6-7 hours a day. Unfortunately it is also the time when the mind is stimulated but not the buttocks, so make sure they don't turn flabby. You need to integrate some cardiovascular exercising, especially those directed towards the gluteal region, i.e. step classes, brisk walking, skipping and running.

In Your Thirties – welcome the baby belly.
A time in life when many women have their children, resulting in flabby stomach muscles that need a little more than breathing in. If you don't work on this area the muscles will just remain lazy and flabby. Remember to ask your doctor's advice if you have recently had a baby.

In Your Forties – welcome sagging arm muscles.
This is the time when muscles in the backs of the arms may begin to follow gravity. To counteract this problem and tone up the muscles, it is important to start exercising the shoulders and arms.

In Your Fifties – welcome thunder thighs.
Although active when younger, with the passing of years motivating one's legs to go for a long walk can get harder but any type of cardiovascular training will remedy this. Try dancing, brisk walking or you're never too old to take up cycling.

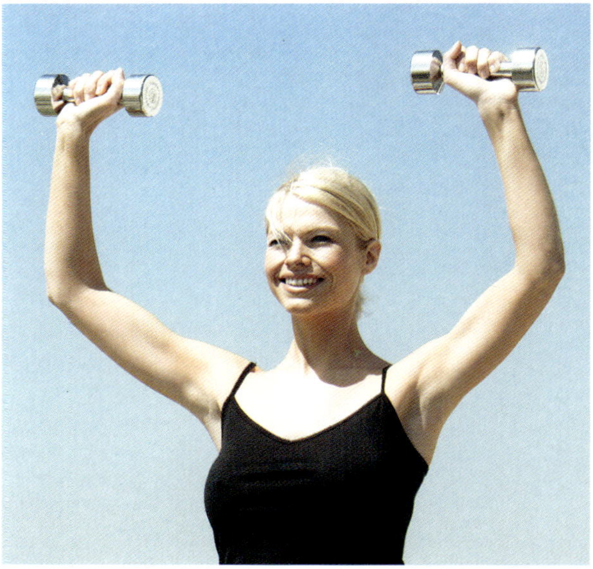

Achieving and maintaining a healthy weight requires a lifelong commitment to healthy eating. The three most important lessons you should have learnt from your programme are to:

✓ Eat a balanced healthy diet
✓ Eat three meals a day
✓ Take some daily exercise